Adrenaline Adventure

Shooting the Curl:
Surfing

Jeff C. Young

ABDO Publishing Company

visit us at
www.abdopublishing.com

Published by ABDO Publishing Company, 8000 West 78th Street, Edina, Minnesota 55439.
Copyright © 2011 by Abdo Consulting Group, Inc. International copyrights reserved in all
countries. No part of this book may be reproduced in any form without written permission from the
publisher. The Checkerboard Library™ is a trademark and logo of ABDO Publishing Company.

Printed in the United States of America, North Mankato, Minnesota.
092010
012011

 PRINTED ON RECYCLED PAPER

Cover Photo: Photolibrary
Interior Photos: Corbis pp. 1, 7, 13, 16–17, 22, 24–25; Getty Images pp. 4–5, 6, 20–21, 28–29;
    iStockphoto p. 11; National Geographic Stock p. 31; Photolibrary pp. 8, 10, 14, 15, 18–19, 27

Series Coordinator: Heidi M.D. Elston
Editors: Heidi M.D. Elston, Megan M. Gunderson
Art Direction & Cover Design: Neil Klinepier

Library of Congress Cataloging-in-Publication Data

Young, Jeff C., 1948-
  Shooting the curl : surfing / Jeff C. Young.
     p. cm. -- (Adrenaline adventure)
  ISBN 978-1-61613-552-2
  1. Surfing--Juvenile literature. I. Title.
  GV839.55.Y68 2011
  797.3'2--dc22

                              2010028242

Contents

Surfing History

People have been riding waves longer than you might think. Many scholars believe surfing started more than 1,000 years ago! Polynesia is generally regarded as the birthplace of surfing. This group of islands lies in the Pacific Ocean.

Surfing also has roots in Hawaii. Early European explorers reported seeing Hawaiians surfing. They described how the native islanders rode the ocean waves on big, wooden boards. Many of the developments in surfing were made in Hawaii.

He'enalu *is the Hawaiian word for "surfing."*

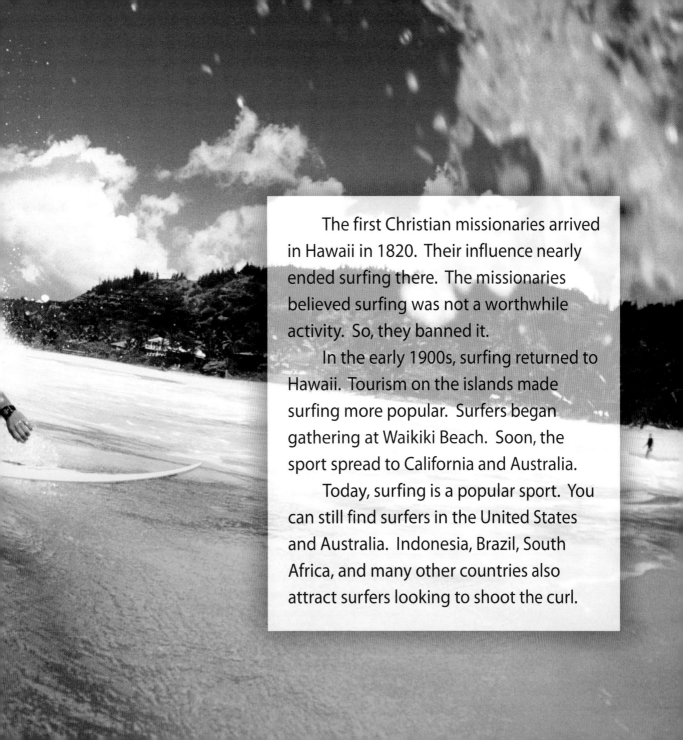

The first Christian missionaries arrived in Hawaii in 1820. Their influence nearly ended surfing there. The missionaries believed surfing was not a worthwhile activity. So, they banned it.

In the early 1900s, surfing returned to Hawaii. Tourism on the islands made surfing more popular. Surfers began gathering at Waikiki Beach. Soon, the sport spread to California and Australia.

Today, surfing is a popular sport. You can still find surfers in the United States and Australia. Indonesia, Brazil, South Africa, and many other countries also attract surfers looking to shoot the curl.

Famous Surfers

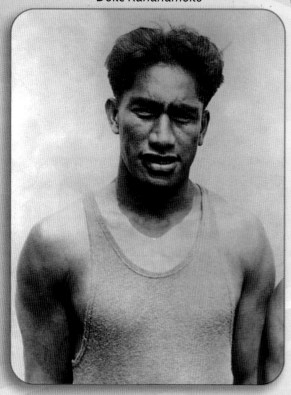

Duke Kahanamoku

In the early 1900s, three surfing pioneers popularized the sport. Duke Kahanamoku was a native Hawaiian and an Olympic champion swimmer. He toured the world giving surfing exhibitions. Thousands came to watch him gracefully ride the waves. Kahanamoku's surfing encouraged and inspired others to take up the sport.

George Freeth was also a top surfer in the early 1900s. Like Kahanamoku, Freeth was from Hawaii. Promoters called him "the Man Who Can Walk on Water." Freeth entertained audiences by standing upright while surfing to the shoreline. He was also one of the first surfers to angle across a wave.

Kelly Slater

Tom Blake changed surfing by making lighter, more **streamlined** surfboards. Blake started making his surfboards in the 1920s. At that time, a typical board weighed between 90 and 150 pounds (40 and 68 kg). Blake made sturdy boards that weighed 40 to 70 pounds (18 to 32 kg). These lighter boards made it possible for more women to surf.

Today, professional surfer Kelly Slater wows crowds with his surfboard skills. Slater won his first world championship title in 1992 at age 20. That year, he became the youngest ever world champion! Slater was 36 when he won his ninth title in 2008. It could be many years before anyone matches or breaks his records.

Surfing Styles

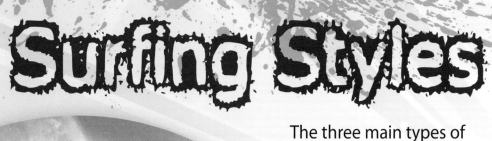

The three main types of surfing are longboarding, shortboarding, and tow-in surfing. All three styles have devoted followers, and all involve catching and riding waves. But, they differ in important ways.

Surfers have used Jet Skis to catch waves more than 30 feet (9 m) high!

Longboarding is a style of surfing that uses boards at least eight feet (2 m) long. It is generally considered a more traditional form of surfing. Longboarding is a smoother, straighter ride. A longboard offers the greatest stability. So, it is the board of choice for smaller waves.

Shortboarding is edgier and more acrobatic than longboarding. Surfers use shorter, lighter boards that are easier to **maneuver** than longboards. Shortboarders can perform tight turns, cutbacks, and aerials. And, they are able to go deeper into the tube of a wave.

In the ocean, the biggest waves break far from shore. Surfers aren't able to paddle fast enough to catch these waves. So, a Jet Ski or a helicopter is used to tow a surfer into a breaking wave.

This style of surfing gives the surfer a running start at catching a large, fast-moving wave. Tow-in surfboards are specially designed for these waves. They come with foot straps, which give the surfer improved balance. Tow-in surfing is very exciting, but it's also very dangerous. Beginning surfers should not attempt it.

Which Board?

Your style of surfing will determine which board best suits your needs. The board you pick should be big enough for you to paddle out easily. It should also be big enough to sit on without sinking.

Every beginning surfer experiences a lot of wipeouts. That's why a lightweight foam board is the best choice for a beginner. It's soft and easy to handle. Getting hit by

When choosing a board, consider a few questions. Does it fit under your arm? Can you carry it? Could you carry it for long distances?

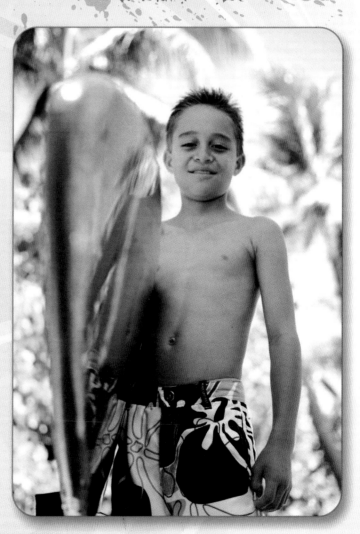

one won't cause a serious injury. With more experience, a beginner can move up to a longboard or a shortboard.

Longboards range in length from 8 to 12 feet (2 to 4 m). They each have one fin attached to the underside. Usually, longboards are the choice of beginning surfers. They offer more stability than shortboards. However because of their size, longboards are more difficult to **maneuver**.

Shortboards are five feet six inches (2 m) or longer and usually have three fins. Shortboards are lighter and thinner than longboards. They are popular with surfers who like to do difficult tricks and quick turns.

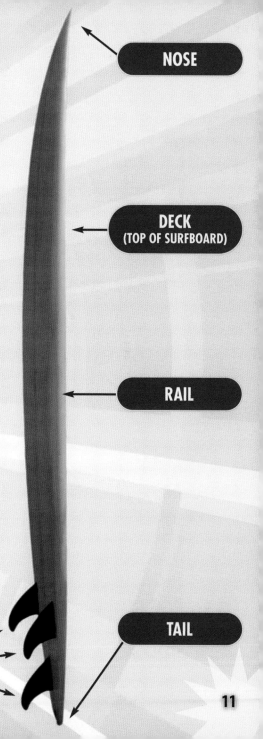

NOSE

DECK
(TOP OF SURFBOARD)

RAIL

TAIL

FINS

Gear Up!

Once you've chosen a board, you'll be eager to start surfing. Still, you need other equipment before you plunge into the water. This additional gear will keep you and other surfers safe.

A surfboard's top surface becomes slippery when wet. For improved **traction**, surfers rub wax on the deck. There are different kinds of waxes for various water temperatures. Surfers use a hard wax in warm water. In mild or cold water, they use a soft wax.

In chilly water, a wet suit will keep you warm. It will also protect you from cuts, scrapes, and sunburn. In water warmer than 75 degrees Fahrenheit (24°C), you could wear a surf shirt instead.

A wipeout can send your board flying! But a leash will keep it from going too far. No more swimming to shore to retrieve your board. The leash also keeps the board from being a danger to other surfers.

It's a good idea to wear a helmet when you surf. A helmet can prevent a head injury during a wipeout. A nose guard for your board is also essential. This rubber bumper fits over your board's nose. The nose guard will protect your board. And, it will reduce injuries to you and other surfers.

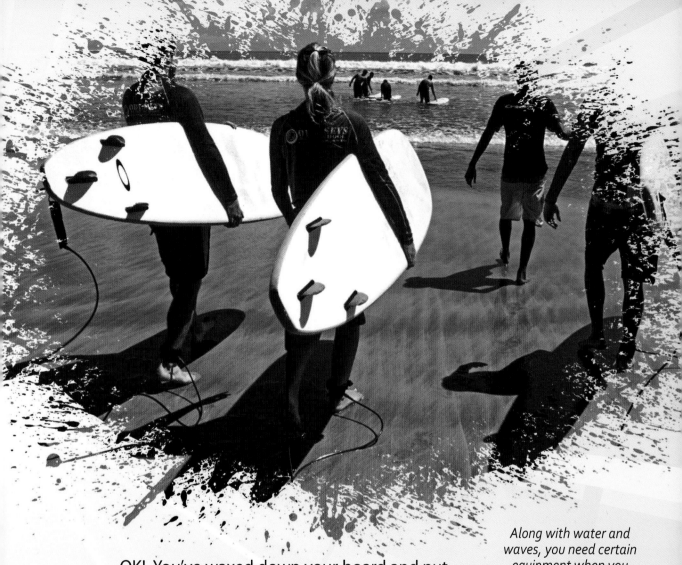

OK! You've waxed down your board and put on your helmet and wet suit. Your nose guard is in place, and you've strapped on your leash. Now you're good to go!

Along with water and waves, you need certain equipment when you surf. Using the right equipment helps protect you from serious injuries.

Let's Surf!

Every beginning surfer needs to master popping up on a surfboard. This gets you from a paddling position to a standing position. Practice popping up on land before heading into the water.

To stand up on your surfboard, grab the rails below your chest and push up. At the same time, move your lower body into a crouched position with one leg forward. This has to be done in one quick, smooth motion.

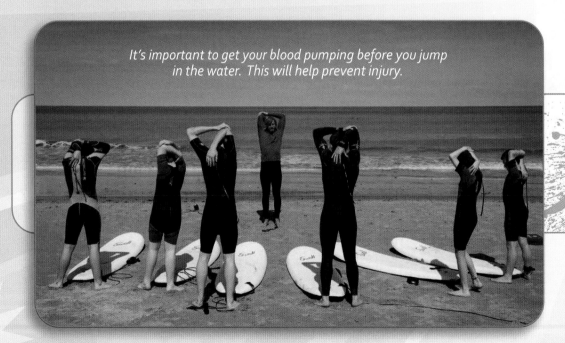

It's important to get your blood pumping before you jump in the water. This will help prevent injury.

How you pop up will show you your **stance**. If you are regular footed, you will stand with your left foot forward. You will stand with your right foot in front if you are goofy footed.

Now, bend your knees slightly. Spread your feet a little farther apart than your shoulders. Stretch out your arms for balance. You're almost ready to get in the water!

First, perform a few stretching exercises. This will warm up the muscles in your arms, legs, back, and shoulders. Surfers that stretch out have fewer injuries. It's also important to get your blood moving. Try walking or jogging on the beach. That way, you will be less likely to get muscle **cramps** in cold water.

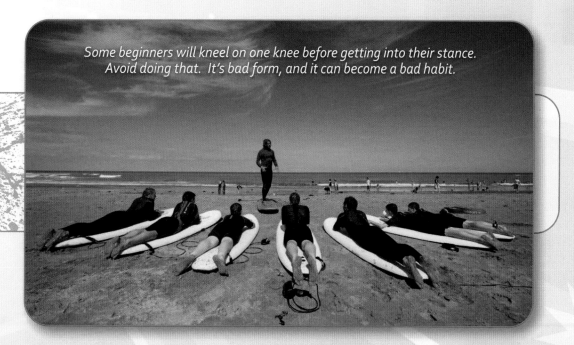

Some beginners will kneel on one knee before getting into their stance. Avoid doing that. It's bad form, and it can become a bad habit.

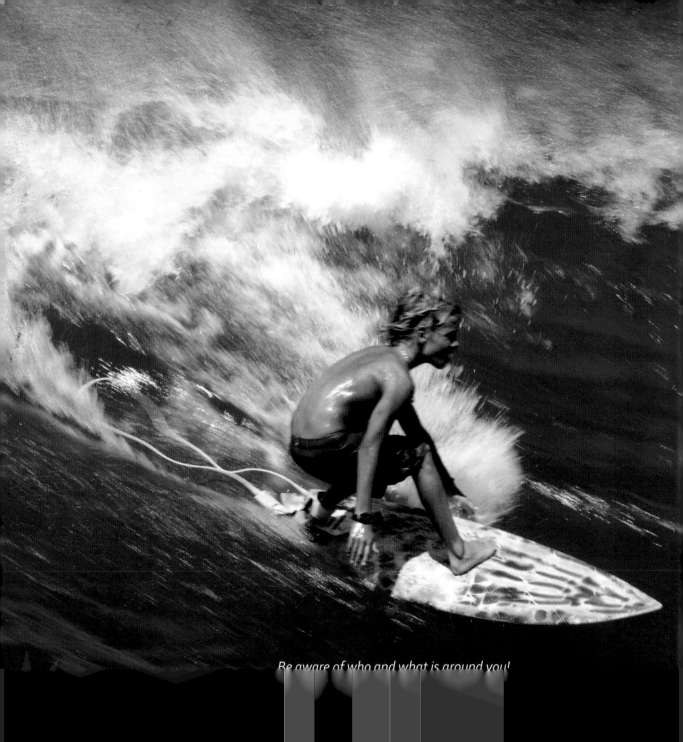

Be aware of who and what is around you!

You've mastered popping up, and you're all stretched out. Now you're ready to paddle out! Lie flat on your board. Keep your weight evenly balanced. If you lie too far forward, the nose will sink. Lie too far back, and the tail will drag.

As a surfer, you'll spend most of your time waiting on waves. Be patient! When you see a wave coming your way, start paddling toward shore. Once the wave starts pushing you forward, stand up. If you're properly balanced, you'll shoot out in front of the breaking wave. Catching your first wave is a moment you will always remember!

Now you can begin learning to turn. Once you can turn, you'll enjoy a longer ride. You turn the board by leaning left or right. This is done by shifting your weight while maintaining your **stance**.

If the wave is breaking from right to left, you'll turn or angle your board to the left. If your wave is breaking from left to right, you'll angle your board to the right. Remember to keep your feet still while shifting your weight. And, use your outstretched arms for balance.

Surfing is like any other sport. The more you practice, the better you will become. Regular practice will build up your strength and **stamina**. You will also gain **confidence**. Don't get discouraged by setbacks. You learned how to walk by falling down. You will learn how to surf by wiping out!

Safe Surfing

Even the most skilled and experienced surfers have accidents and suffer injuries. Using safety equipment such as helmets and leashes will make surfing safer for you. But these items alone won't prevent accidents. You must also follow some common safety practices.

The ocean may look like a calm, peaceful place. But, it can be violent and **unpredictable**. That's why you should never surf alone. Use the buddy system! That way, someone will be nearby to help if you run into trouble. Also, don't try to ride a bigger wave than you can handle. Accidents occur when surfers overestimate their abilities.

Every surfer wipes out. Learning to fall safely can prevent a serious injury.

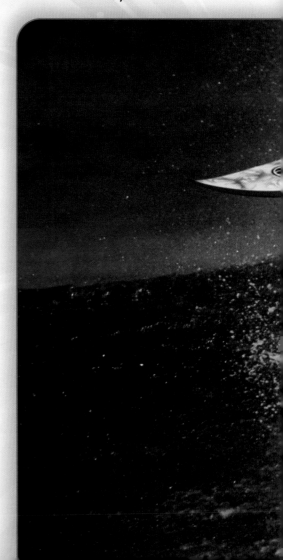

When wiping out, kick your board in front of you. If that's not possible, push the board to the side. When you come up for air, cover your head with your arms. This will help protect your head if you're not wearing a helmet.

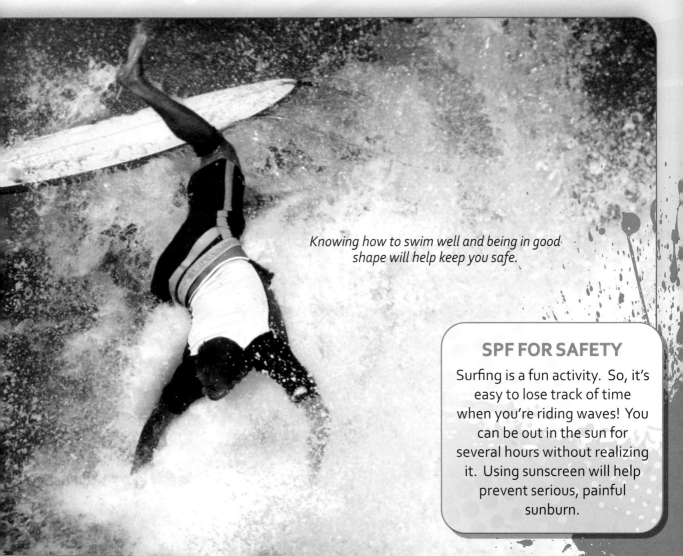

Knowing how to swim well and being in good shape will help keep you safe.

SPF FOR SAFETY

Surfing is a fun activity. So, it's easy to lose track of time when you're riding waves! You can be out in the sun for several hours without realizing it. Using sunscreen will help prevent serious, painful sunburn.

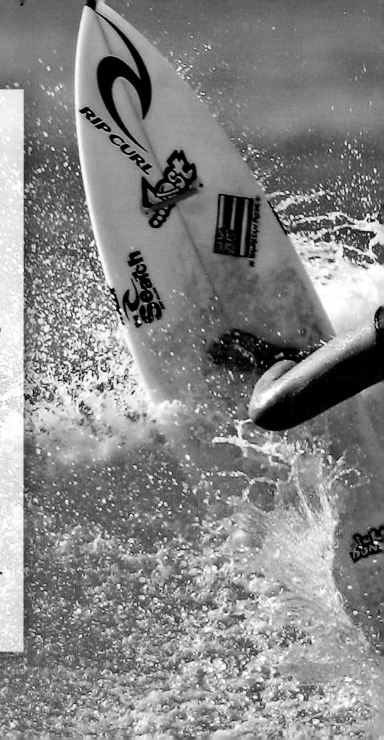

Sometimes, surfing accidents occur from natural hazards. These include **rip currents**, marine animals, and underwater reefs and rocks. It's important to know how to handle such unexpected dangers.

If you get caught in a rip current, don't try to swim against it. Swim in the direction where you feel the least resistance. Usually, this will be in a direction parallel to the shore.

Jellyfish and sharks are two marine animals that surfers need to watch out for. Jellyfish can give painful stings. Sometimes, sharks

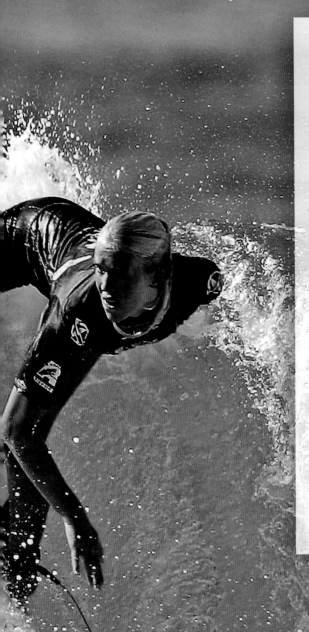

In 2003, 13-year-old surfer Bethany Hamilton was attacked by a shark off the coast of Hawaii. The shark bit off her arm at the shoulder. Still, she was back in the water after just a few months. Today, Hamilton is proving to be a rising star in the surfing world.

mistake surfers for sea animals such as seals and attack.

There are several ways to avoid sharks. Surf at beaches with lots of people and noise. Avoid surfing near fishing boats or seal colonies. Sharks swim around those places to look for food. Sharks are also attracted to blood. So, stay out of the water if you're bleeding or have an open wound.

The safest surfers learn about a surfing spot before they get in the water. They find places where there aren't any underwater reefs or rocks. If a spot looks deserted, it might be for a reason. If there are lifeguards nearby, ask them if the spot is safe for surfing.

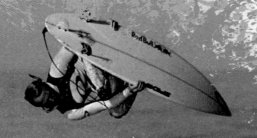

In order to compete, NSSA members must earn good grades in school.

Competition

    While surfing is fun, it's also a competitive sport. Ever since Hawaiians began surfing, there have been contests to determine the best surfers. Today, the best professionals can earn a good income.

The Association of Surfing Professionals (ASP) is the governing body of professional surfing. It has six professional surfing **circuits**. These include the ASP World Tour, the World Qualifying Series, and the World Longboard Tour. The ASP also runs the Pro Junior Series, the World Masters Championship, and Specialty Events.

All professional surfers want to be on the ASP World Tour! It includes both men's and women's divisions. Surfers compete for money and the ASP world title.

Surfing competitions aren't just for professionals. The International Surfing Association (ISA) governs the sport of surfing. Each year, the ISA holds the World Surfing Games. This is one of the largest competitive surfing events in the world. The ISA also **sponsors** many other competitions throughout the world. And, it is working to get surfing included in the Olympic Games.

The National Scholastic Surfing Association (NSSA) promotes surfing for students. The NSSA is the leading amateur competitive surfing organization in the United States.

In most surfing contests, four surfers at a time compete in **heats**. Each heat can last up to 30 minutes. Surfers try to ride waves as long as possible while performing various **maneuvers**.

Usually, the surfers are judged by their four best waves. The top two surfers in each **heat** advance to the next round.

Judges grade competitors in four different categories. The first is the quality of the **maneuvers**. Second is how close the surfer gets to the curl of the wave while performing them. Third, judges determine the level of difficulty of the wave the surfer is riding. And finally, judges time how long the surfer rides the wave.

Judges give top marks to surfers who take the biggest risks. They look for radical, controlled maneuvers. These include floaters, aerials, tube rides, and cutbacks. The judges also look for power and speed. They reward points based on quality.

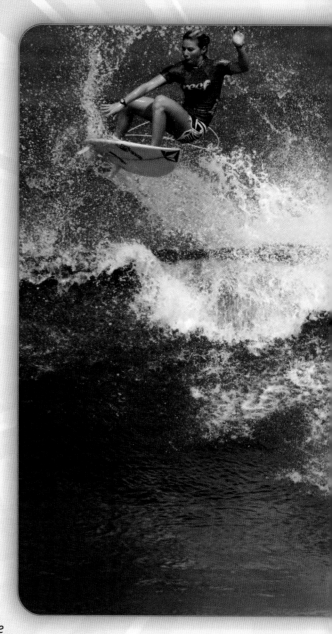

Competitive surfers need to be creative and daring to win over the judges.

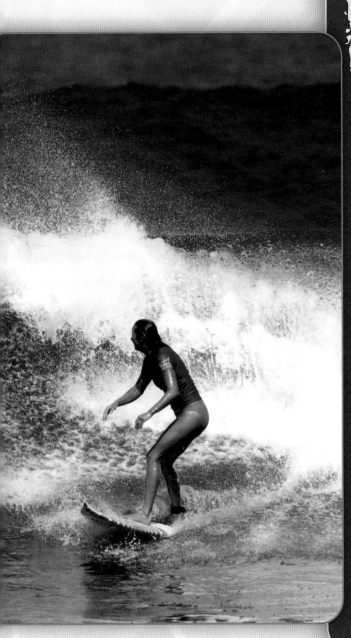

LINGO

AERIAL – an acrobatic maneuver performed in the air.

CUTBACK – a 180-degree turn that is done on either of the two edges of the surfboard. It allows the surfer to be positioned toward the breaking part of the wave.

FLOATER – floating the board along the top of a breaking wave.

GNARLY – an intense or dangerous thing, person, or situation.

GREMMIE OR **GROMMET** – a young surfer.

GUN – a big-wave surfboard.

HANG TEN – a longboarding maneuver. The rider hangs all ten toes off the surfboard's nose.

HOTDOGGING – fancy or trick surfing.

SOUP – the white water from a breaking wave.

STOKED – excited, pleased, happy, thrilled.

TUBE RIDE – when a surfer rides through the tunnel formed by a hollow, breaking wave.

WAVE HOG – someone who won't share a wave.

WIPEOUT – a ride-ending mishap.

Respect Others

As surfing has become more popular, beaches have grown more crowded. To keep things orderly, surfers have a code of conduct. All surfers must obey a few common sense rules. This will help them make new friends and earn the respect of other surfers.

First, never drop in on a wave in front of another surfer. Second, the first surfer on the wave always has the right-of-way. Third, the surfer closest to the breaking part of the wave has the right-of-way.

These important rules are all about yielding the right-of-way. In short, if someone is already riding a wave, stay out of his or her way. If you're paddling out, stay clear of incoming surfers.

Another important rule is that surfers look out for each other. If you see a surfer in trouble, alert other surfers in the area. Be willing to stop surfing to come to the aid of another surfer.

Never try to knock another surfer off of his or her board. This could cause a serious injury. Other surfers won't put up with such behavior.

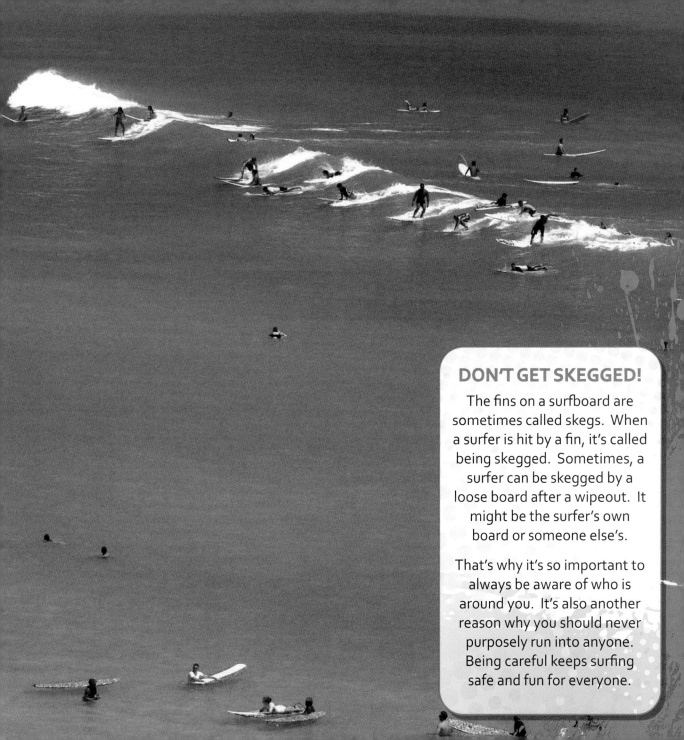

DON'T GET SKEGGED!

The fins on a surfboard are sometimes called skegs. When a surfer is hit by a fin, it's called being skegged. Sometimes, a surfer can be skegged by a loose board after a wipeout. It might be the surfer's own board or someone else's.

That's why it's so important to always be aware of who is around you. It's also another reason why you should never purposely run into anyone. Being careful keeps surfing safe and fun for everyone.

Catch a Wave!

    Almost anyone can learn to surf. First, you must be a strong swimmer and be in good shape. Know the safety practices and rules before taking to the waves. Then, find a friend or a relative who surfs to teach you. Or, look for a qualified instructor or a surfing school.

    For a beginner, the best place to learn to surf is a spot with slow, gentle waves. You'll have time to read the waves and study how they break. You'll also be able to work on your form.

    Several of the best surfing areas in the United States are found in California. They include Malibu and Huntington Beach. The East Coast is popular, too. Favorite spots include Atlantic City, New Jersey, and Cape Hatteras, North Carolina. In Hawaii, Waikiki, Waimea Bay, and Sunset Beach are some of the best-known places to surf.

Using the buddy system keeps surfing fun and safe!

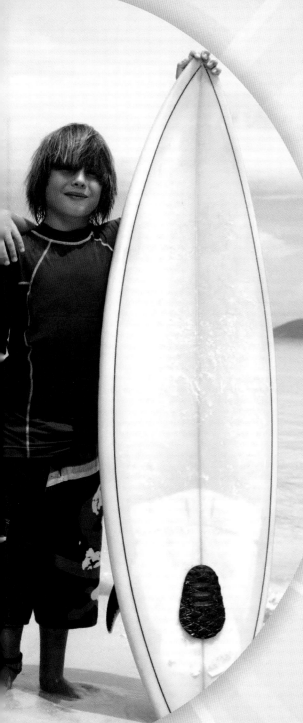

Surfing magazine named Kirra, Australia, one of the "Ten Best Waves in the World." The high-quality waves around Biarritz, France, have been the site of many world surfing competitions. Brazil's 5,000 miles (8,000 km) of Atlantic coastline also provide many popular surfing spots.

Surfing has physical benefits when you do it regularly. There are also mental and social advantages. Surfing relaxes you and gives you a break from your worries and cares. And, interacting with other surfers gives you a chance to increase your circle of friends. With enough practice, you'll soon be shooting the curl!

Glossary

circuit - an association or league of sports teams.

confidence - faith in oneself and one's powers.

cramp - a sharp, painful tightening that occurs suddenly in a muscle.

heat - a single trial in a contest used to determine which competitors will compete in the finals.

maneuver (muh-NOO-vuhr) - to make changes in direction and position for a specific purpose. A maneuver is a clever or skillful move or action.

rip current - a strong current of water flowing outward from the shore.

sponsor - to finance an event.

stamina - the power to endure fatigue, disease, or hardship.

stance - a way of standing or being placed.

streamlined - designed to offer the least possible resistance when moving through air or water.

traction - friction between a body and the surface on which it moves. Traction enables the body to move without slipping.

unpredictable - unable to be guessed or declared in advance.

Web Sites

To learn more about surfing, visit ABDO Publishing Company online. Web sites about surfing are featured on our Book Links page. These links are routinely monitored and updated to provide the most current information available.
www.abdopublishing.com

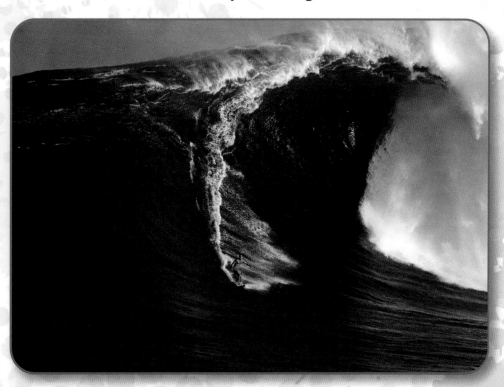

Index